WHEN IS THE BEST TIME TO WORKOUT

OLUSEGUN SETH AJULO

TABLE OF CONTENT

INTRODUCTION

The best time to work out varies for each person and depends on individual preferences, schedule, and goals. Some people prefer morning workouts to kickstart their day, while others find evening sessions more convenient after work. Ultimately, the best time to work out is when you can consistently commit to your fitness routine, ensuring regular exercise and overall well-being.

IMPORTANCE OF REGULAR EXERCISE

Regular exercise offers a multitude of benefits for both physical and mental health. It helps improve cardiovascular health, strengthen muscles and bones, enhance flexibility, and boost overall energy levels. Exercise also plays a crucial role in managing body weight, reducing the risk of chronic diseases such as diabetes and heart disease, and improving immune function.

Beyond physical health, regular exercise has significant mental health advantages. It reduces stress, anxiety, and depression by promoting the release of endorphins, which are natural mood lifters. Exercise can also improve sleep quality, increase cognitive function, and enhance self-esteem and body image.

Incorporating regular physical activity into one's routine can lead to a healthier, happier life, making it an essential component of overall well-being.

DEBUNKING COMMON MYTHS ABOUT WORKOUT TIMING

Here are a few common myths about workout timing debunked:

Myth 1: Morning workouts are the only effective ones.

Debunked: The best time to work out depends on your personal preference and schedule. Whether you exercise in the morning, afternoon, or evening, consistency and commitment are key to achieving your fitness goals.

Myth 2: Exercising on an empty stomach burns more fat.

Debunked: While fasted cardio can lead to burning a slightly higher percentage of calories from fat, the overall calorie burn matters more for weight loss. Eating a balanced meal before exercise can provide energy, enhance performance, and prevent muscle loss.

Myth 3: You shouldn't eat after a workout if you want to lose weight.

Debunked: Post-workout nutrition is crucial for recovery. Consuming a combination of protein and carbohydrates helps repair muscles, replenish glycogen stores, and supports overall recovery. It doesn't necessarily lead to weight gain if you stay within your daily calorie limit.

Myth 4: Cardio is the only way to lose weight; strength training makes you bulky.

Debunked: Both cardio and strength training are essential. Cardio helps burn calories and improve cardiovascular health, while strength training builds lean muscle mass, boosts metabolism, and enhances overall body composition. Strength training doesn't automatically make you bulky; it depends on your training approach and nutrition.

Myth 5: Exercising sporadically is enough to stay fit.

Debunked: Consistency is key to fitness. Regular, consistent exercise is more effective than sporadic, intense workouts. It's important to establish a sustainable routine that you can maintain over the long term to see lasting results in your fitness journey.

UNDERSTANDING CARCADIAN RHYTHMS

Circadian rhythms are the body's internal biological clocks that regulate various physiological processes, such as sleep-wake cycles, body temperature, hormone secretion, and metabolism. These rhythms follow a roughly 24-hour cycle and are influenced by external cues like light and darkness.

The suprachiasmatic nucleus (SCN) in the brain's hypothalamus acts as the master clock, receiving signals from the eyes about light and darkness. This information helps synchronize the body's internal clocks with the external environment. Circadian rhythms influence not only sleep patterns but also hormone release, hunger, and other bodily functions.

Understanding circadian

Circadian rhythms are biological cycles that repeat approximately every 24 hours. These rhythms are found in most living organisms, including animals, plants, and even some bacteria. They regulate various physiological and behavioral processes, such as sleep-wake patterns, hormone secretion, body temperature, and metabolism.

The key component regulating circadian rhythms is the suprachiasmatic nucleus (SCN) in the brain, often referred to as the body's master clock. The SCN receives information about light and darkness from the eyes, helping it align the body's internal clocks with the natural light-dark cycle. This synchronization is crucial for maintaining a consistent sleep-wake cycle and other bodily functions.

EXPLANATION OF CIRCADIAN RHYTHMS AND THEIR IMPACT ON THE BODY

1. Sleep-Wake Cycle: Circadian rhythms play a significant role in determining when you feel alert and when you feel sleepy. Disruptions to these rhythms, such as shift work or jet lag, can lead to sleep disorders and overall fatigue.

2. Hormone Regulation: Circadian rhythms influence the release of hormones like cortisol, which is associated with wakefulness, and melatonin, which promotes sleep. Proper regulation of these hormones is essential for overall health.

3. Metabolism: Circadian rhythms affect the body's metabolic processes, including the regulation of appetite, digestion, and energy expenditure. Irregular eating patterns or disrupted circadian rhythms can contribute to metabolic disorders and weight gain.

4. Cognitive Function: Circadian rhythms can impact cognitive abilities such as memory, attention, and alertness. Disruptions in these rhythms may affect mental clarity and focus.

5. Mood and Emotional Well-Being: Imbalances in circadian rhythms have been linked to mood disorders such as depression and bipolar disorder. Maintaining regular sleep patterns and exposure to natural light can help regulate mood.

Overall, a consistent daily routine that aligns with natural light-dark cycles can support healthy circadian rhythms. This includes maintaining regular sleep schedules, getting exposure to natural light during the day, and avoiding bright artificial light, especially blue light, close to bedtime. Properly regulated circadian rhythms contribute to overall well-being and can positively impact various aspects of physical and mental health.

HOW CIRCADIAN RHYTHMS AFFECT ENERGY LEVELS AND PERFORMANCE

Circadian rhythms have a significant impact on energy levels and performance throughout the day. Here's how:

1. Energy Levels: Circadian rhythms influence the body's natural energy peaks and dips. Typically, energy levels are highest during the late morning and early afternoon, corresponding to the body's natural waking period. During these times, cognitive functions, alertness, and physical performance tend to be at their peak. Energy levels dip during the late afternoon, often referred to as the "afternoon slump," and then rise again in the early evening.

2. Performance: Cognitive and physical performance tend to be optimized during the body's peak energy periods. For instance, reaction times, memory retention, and problem-solving skills are generally better during the late morning and early afternoon. Physical performance, including strength, endurance, and coordination, also tends to be at its best during these times.

Disruptions to circadian rhythms, such as irregular sleep patterns, jet lag, or shift work, can significantly impact energy levels and performance. Shift workers, for example, often experience reduced alertness and impaired cognitive function due to misaligned circadian rhythms.

Additionally, the timing of meals and physical activity can influence how circadian rhythms affect energy and performance. Eating meals at consistent times and engaging in regular exercise can help synchronize the body's internal clocks, leading to more stable energy levels and better performance.

In summary, circadian rhythms regulate energy levels and performance by influencing the body's natural peaks and dips in alertness and cognitive/physical abilities throughout the day. Maintaining a consistent sleep schedule, regular meal times, and incorporating physical activity can help optimize energy levels and performance by keeping circadian rhythms in sync.

MORNING WORKOUTS: PROS AND CONS

Here are the pros and cons of morning workouts:

Pros:

1. Consistency: Exercising in the morning helps establish a routine as there are fewer interruptions and distractions compared to later in the day. It can lead to greater consistency in your fitness regimen.

2. Boosts Metabolism: Morning workouts kickstart your metabolism, helping you burn more calories throughout the day. This can be beneficial for weight management and overall energy balance.

3. Enhanced Focus and Productivity: Exercise releases endorphins, which can improve mood and increase focus. Starting your day with a workout might enhance your productivity and mental clarity.

4. Better Sleep: Regular morning exercise has been linked to improved sleep quality. It can help regulate your sleep-wake cycle, leading to more restful nights.

5. Sense of Accomplishment: Completing a workout in the morning gives you a sense of accomplishment early in the day, setting a positive tone for the rest of your activities.

Cons:

1. Early Wake-Up: Morning workouts require waking up early, which might be challenging for night owls or people with irregular sleep patterns. Insufficient sleep can negatively impact exercise performance and recovery.

2. Body Temperature and Flexibility: Body temperature is usually lower in the morning, which might increase the risk of injuries if not properly warmed up. It might take longer for your body to reach its optimal flexibility and performance levels.

3. Crowded Gym: Many individuals prefer working out in the morning, leading to crowded gyms during peak hours. This could mean longer wait times for equipment or limited space for certain exercises.

4. Nutrition Timing: It might be challenging to have a pre-workout meal if you're not accustomed to eating early in the morning. Proper nutrition before a workout can affect your energy levels and performance.

5. Scheduling Constraints: Morning workouts might not align with everyone's schedule, especially for those with early work commitments, family responsibilities, or other obligations.

BENEFITS OF MORNING WORKOUTS

Ultimately, whether morning workouts are suitable for you depends on your personal preferences, lifestyle, and body's natural rhythms. It's essential to find a workout time that fits your schedule and allows you to be consistent and enjoy your fitness routine.

Morning workouts can indeed have a positive impact on metabolism. Here's how:

1. Increased Resting Metabolic Rate: Regular physical activity, especially in the morning, can increase your resting metabolic rate (RMR). RMR is the number of calories your body needs to maintain basic physiological functions while at rest. By boosting your RMR, you burn more calories throughout the day, aiding in weight management.

2. Enhanced Caloric Burn: Morning workouts kickstart your metabolism, causing your body to burn calories for energy. This effect can last for several hours after the workout, leading to an overall increase in daily caloric expenditure.

3. Improved Insulin Sensitivity: Exercise, particularly in the morning, improves insulin sensitivity. Enhanced insulin sensitivity means your body can more effectively regulate blood sugar levels. This can reduce the risk of developing type 2 diabetes and help with weight management.

4. Preservation of Lean Muscle Mass: Morning workouts, especially those that include strength training, help preserve and build lean muscle mass. Muscles burn more calories at rest compared to fat tissue. By increasing your muscle mass, you enhance your body's ability to burn calories throughout the day, even when you're not exercising.

5. Optimal Hormonal Balance: Exercise in the morning helps regulate hormones related to metabolism and appetite, such as cortisol and ghrelin. Proper balance of these hormones can support a healthy metabolism and prevent overeating.

6. Establishing a Routine: Morning workouts often become a consistent part of your daily routine. Regularity in physical activity can positively impact metabolism over time, making it easier for your body to maintain a healthy weight.

It's important to note that the benefits of morning workouts on metabolism are not solely dependent on the time of day you exercise. The key is to engage in regular physical activity, whether in the morning, afternoon, or evening, to experience these metabolic advantages. Choosing a workout time that fits your schedule and allows for consistency is crucial for long-term success in boosting metabolism and overall health.

ENHANCING MENTAL CLARITY AND FOCUS

Enhancing mental clarity and focus involves adopting various strategies that promote cognitive function and reduce distractions. Here are some effective methods to improve mental clarity and focus:

1. Regular Exercise: Physical activity increases blood flow to the brain, promoting the growth of new brain cells and enhancing overall cognitive function. Aim for regular aerobic exercises, which have been shown to improve memory and attention.

2. Adequate Sleep: Quality sleep is essential for mental clarity and focus. Lack of sleep can impair cognitive abilities, attention, and decision-making. Aim for 7-9 hours of sleep per night to ensure your brain functions optimally.

3. Healthy Diet: A balanced diet rich in antioxidants, vitamins, and omega-3 fatty acids supports brain health. Foods like fish, nuts, fruits, and vegetables are known to enhance cognitive function. Avoid excessive sugar and processed foods, as they can lead to energy crashes and brain fog.

4. Stress Management: Chronic stress can impair concentration and mental clarity. Practice relaxation techniques such as deep breathing, meditation, yoga, or mindfulness to manage stress levels effectively.

5. Stay Hydrated: Dehydration can lead to fatigue, headaches, and decreased cognitive abilities. Drink an adequate amount of water throughout the day to maintain optimal brain function.

6. Mindfulness and Meditation: These practices can improve focus, attention, and overall cognitive flexibility. Regular mindfulness meditation has been shown to enhance the ability to sustain attention on a specific task.

7. Limit Distractions: Create a focused work environment by minimizing distractions. Turn off notifications, designate specific time slots for tasks, and establish a dedicated workspace to enhance concentration.

8. Break Tasks into Smaller Steps: Breaking tasks into smaller, manageable steps can prevent feeling overwhelmed and improve focus on completing one task at a time.

9. Regular Breaks: Taking short breaks during work or study sessions can actually improve productivity. Brief periods of rest or physical activity can rejuvenate the brain, leading to better focus when you return to the task.

10. Challenge Your Brain: Engage in activities that challenge your brain, such as puzzles, learning a new skill, or reading. Mental stimulation can improve cognitive function and enhance focus.

By incorporating these practices into your daily routine, you can enhance your mental clarity, focus, and overall cognitive abilities, leading to improved productivity and well-being.

CHALLENGES OF MORNING WORKOUTS

Warming up your body effectively is crucial for preventing injuries and optimizing performance during morning workouts. Here are some challenges associated with warming up in the morning and how to overcome them:

Challenge 1: Morning Stiffness

In the morning, your body might feel stiff due to the lack of movement during sleep. This stiffness can make it challenging to perform dynamic movements during warm-up exercises.

Solution: Start your warm-up with gentle, low-impact exercises. Focus on mobility exercises that target major joints like shoulders, hips, and ankles. Perform slow and controlled movements to gradually increase your range of motion.

Challenge 2: Low Body Temperature

Your body temperature is lower in the morning, which can affect muscle flexibility and increase the risk of injury if you jump into intense exercises without proper warming up.

Solution: Begin your warm-up with light aerobic activities like brisk walking, jogging in place, or cycling. These activities gradually increase your heart rate and body temperature, preparing your muscles for more dynamic stretches and exercises.

Challenge 3: Time Constraints

Morning workouts are often done before work or other daily responsibilities, so there might be limited time to dedicate to a lengthy warm-up routine.

Solution: opt for a focused warm-up routine that targets key muscle groups. Choose dynamic stretches that engage multiple muscle groups simultaneously. Perform exercises like leg swings, arm circles, bodyweight squats, and lunges, which effectively warm up various muscle groups in a short amount of time.

Challenge 4: Lack of Energy

In the morning, you might feel groggy or low on energy, making it difficult to engage in a vigorous warm-up.

Solution: Start your warm-up with deep breathing exercises and gentle stretches to awaken your body and mind. Gradually progress to more dynamic movements as you begin to feel more awake and energized.

Challenge 5: Cold Environment

During certain seasons, the morning environment can be chilly, making it uncomfortable to warm up the body effectively.

Solution: Dress in layers to keep your muscles warm. Begin your warm-up indoors if possible, and gradually transition to outdoor exercises. Engage in bodyweight exercises that generate internal heat, such as jumping jacks or high knees, to warm up quickly.

By addressing these challenges with appropriate warm-up strategies, you can prepare your body effectively for morning workouts, reducing the risk of injuries and ensuring a more productive exercise session.

BALANCING WORKOUT ROUTINE WITH MORNING ROUTINE

Balancing your workout routine with your morning routine requires planning and consistency. Here are a few tips to help you achieve a balanced routine:

1. Set a Schedule: Determine a specific time slot in the morning for your workouts. This could be before work or any other commitments. Consistency is key.

2. Prepare the Night Before: Lay out your workout clothes and any necessary equipment the night before. This saves time and makes it easier to get started in the morning.

3. Start with Short Workouts: If you're new to morning workouts, start with short and manageable exercises. As you get used to the routine, you can gradually increase the duration and intensity.

4. Include Varlety: Incorporate different types of exercises to keep your routine interesting. This can include cardio, strength training, flexibility exercises, or even yoga.

5. Plan Efficient Workouts: Opt for high-intensity interval training (HIIT) or other time-efficient workout routines. These can be very effective and take less time compared to traditional workouts.

6. Prioritize Sleep: Ensure you are getting enough sleep to wake up feeling refreshed and motivated for your morning workout. Quality sleep is crucial for recovery and overall well-being.

7. Stay Hydrated and Fuel Your Body: Drink water and have a light snack before your workout to provide your body with the necessary energy. After the workout, have a balanced breakfast to refuel.

8. Be Flexible: Life can be unpredictable. If you miss a morning workout, don't be too hard on yourself. Adapt your schedule and find another time during the day to fit in some physical activity.

Remember, finding the right balance takes time and experimentation. Listen to your body and adjust your routine accordingly to make it sustainable in the long run.

AFTERNOON WORKOUTS: PROS AND CONS

Here are the pros and cons of afternoon workouts:

Pros:

1. Increased Body Temperature: Your body temperature naturally peaks in the late afternoon, which can lead to better physical performance and reduced risk of injury.

2. Improved Physical Performance: Strength, speed, and endurance tend to be at their peak in the late afternoon, making it an optimal time for intense workouts.

3. Reduced Risk of Injury: Warmer muscles and joints are more flexible and less prone to injury, allowing for a more effective and safer workout session.

4. Better Mental Focus: By the afternoon, your mind is usually more alert and focused, enabling you to engage in your workout routine with greater concentration and determination.

5. Opportunity for Social Activities: Afternoon workouts can be a social activity, allowing you to exercise with friends or attend group classes, providing motivation and accountability.

6. Stress Relief: Afternoon workouts can help alleviate stress accumulated during the day, providing a healthy way to unwind and boost your mood

Cons:

1. Schedule Constraints: Busy work or school schedules might make it difficult to find a consistent time for afternoon workouts, leading to irregular exercise habits.

2. Crowded Gyms: If you prefer working out at a gym, afternoons can be a peak time, resulting in crowded facilities and potential wait times for equipment.

3. Energy Fluctuations: Some people experience energy dips in the late afternoon, making it challenging to find the motivation to work out after a long day.

4. Evening Commitments: Social events, family obligations, or other evening activities might interfere with your ability to establish a regular afternoon workout routine.

5. Potential Disruptions: Afternoons can be unpredictable, and unexpected events or work-related tasks might arise, disrupting your planned workout session.

6. Body Temperature Variability: While body temperature peaks in the late afternoon for most people, individual variations exist, and this peak might occur at different times for some individuals.

Ultimately, the best time for a workout depends on your personal schedule, energy levels, and preferences. Finding a consistent time that fits into your routine and allows you to stay committed to your fitness goals is key, whether it's in the morning, afternoon, or evening.

BENEFITS OF AFTERNOON WORKOUTS

Afternoon workouts offer distinct benefits related to peak muscle strength and flexibility:

1. Peak Muscle Strength: In the afternoon, your body temperature tends to be higher, which can enhance muscle flexibility and reduce the risk of injuries. Higher body temperature also improves muscle function, allowing you to lift heavier weights and engage in more intense strength training exercises. This increased muscle strength can lead to more effective resistance training and overall muscle development.

2. Improved Flexibility: Warmer muscles are more pliable and less prone to strains and sprains. Engaging in flexibility exercises, such as yoga or stretching routines, during the afternoon can lead to greater gains in overall flexibility. Improved flexibility not only enhances athletic performance but also supports better posture and reduces the likelihood of muscle imbalances and injuries.

By capitalizing on the body's natural circadian rhythms and taking advantage of the increased body temperature in the afternoon, you can optimize your workouts to achieve better muscle strength and flexibility. This can lead to more efficient training sessions and overall improvements in physical fitness.

INCREASED CARDIOVASCULAR PERFORMANCE

Engaging in afternoon workouts can lead to increased cardiovascular performance. Here's how:

1. Optimal Body Temperature: In the afternoon, your body temperature is higher, which means your muscles are warmer and more flexible. This warm-up effect reduces the resistance in your cardiovascular system, allowing for easier blood flow to the muscles. As a result, your heart doesn't have to work as hard to deliver oxygen and nutrients to the muscles, improving overall cardiovascular efficiency.

2. Improved Endurance: With the body at an optimal temperature in the afternoon, you're likely to experience better endurance during cardiovascular exercises such as running, cycling, or swimming. Your muscles can work more efficiently, allowing you to sustain activities for longer periods and achieve greater cardiovascular benefits.

3. Enhanced Oxygen Uptake: Warmer muscles and increased blood flow mean that your body can take in oxygen more effectively. This improved oxygen uptake benefits your cardiovascular system by enhancing the efficiency of your heart and lungs. Your body can deliver oxygen to working muscles more efficiently, allowing for better aerobic performance.

4. Consistent Performance: By the afternoon, your body has typically fully recovered from the morning's activities and is ready for another bout of exercise. This can lead to more consistent and effective cardiovascular workouts, as your body is primed for physical activity.

5. Better Hydration and Nutrition: Throughout the day, you've likely had the opportunity to hydrate and fuel your body with nutritious meals and snacks. Proper hydration and nutrition are essential for optimal cardiovascular performance, ensuring that your body has the necessary resources to sustain physical activity.

Incorporating cardiovascular exercises into your afternoon routine can take advantage of these factors, leading to improved cardiovascular performance, endurance, and overall fitness levels. Remember to stay hydrated, warm up properly, and listen to your body to maximize the benefits of your afternoon workouts.

CHALLENGES OF AFTERNOON WORKOUTS

FINDING MOTIVATION AFTER A LONG DAY

Finding motivation for afternoon workouts after a long day can indeed be challenging. Here are some strategies to overcome this hurdle:

1. Create a Routine: Establish a consistent workout schedule in the afternoon. By making exercise a daily habit at the same time, it becomes easier to find motivation as your body and mind adapt to the routine.

2. Accountability: Exercise with a friend or join a group fitness class. Having a workout buddy or being part of a community provides accountability and makes the experience more enjoyable, motivating you to show up even after a tiring day.

3. Set Clear Goals: Define specific, achievable fitness goals. Whether it's improving endurance, losing weight, or building strength, having clear objectives can give you a sense of purpose and motivation to work out, even on challenging days.

4. Reward Yourself: Treat yourself after a successful workout. It could be a relaxing bath, your favorite snack, or watching an episode of your favorite TV show. Knowing there's a reward waiting can provide the extra push you need.

5. Choose Enjoyable Activities: Engage in exercises you genuinely enjoy. Whether it's dancing, cycling, or practicing martial arts, doing something you love increases the likelihood of staying motivated and committed.

6. Visualize Benefits: Remind yourself of the benefits of exercising, such as increased energy, stress relief, and improved mood. Visualizing these positive outcomes can boost your motivation to lace up your workout shoes.

7. Break It Down: If the idea of a long workout feels daunting, break it into smaller, manageable segments. Short, intense workouts or split routines throughout the day can be just as effective and less overwhelming.

8. Mindset Shift: Instead of viewing exercise as a chore, reframe it as a way to unwind and de-stress. Think of it as "me time" where you can focus on yourself and your well-being.

9. Morning Prep: Pack your gym bag or lay out your workout clothes in the morning. Having everything ready reduces friction and makes it easier to get started when you come home.

10. Be Kind to Yourself: Understand that some days, despite your best efforts, you might not feel up to working out. Don't be too hard on yourself; listen to your body and consider taking a rest day if needed. Consistency is essential, but so is self-compassion.

Finding the right motivation might take time, so experiment with these strategies to discover what works best for you. Remember that every effort counts, and taking small steps toward your fitness goals is a significant achievement.

MANAGING POST-LUNCH ENERGY LEVELS

Managing post-lunch energy levels is crucial for staying productive and focused throughout the day. Here are some tips to help you maintain your energy levels after lunch:

1. Balanced Lunch: Opt for a balanced meal that includes protein, complex carbohydrates, and healthy fats. Avoid heavy, carb-laden lunches that can lead to energy crashes. Include vegetables, lean proteins, whole grains, and good fats like those found in avocados or nuts.

2. Stay Hydrated: Dehydration can cause fatigue. Drink water throughout the day to stay hydrated. Consider having a cup of herbal tea or infused water for variety.

3. Mindful Eating: Eat slowly and mindfully. Chew your food thoroughly, savoring each bite. This not only aids digestion but also gives your body time to register that it's full, preventing overeating and energy slumps.

4. Avoid Sugary Snacks: While sugar might provide a quick energy boost, it's often followed by a crash. Opt for healthier snacks like fruits, nuts, or yogurt to maintain stable blood sugar levels.

5. Take Short Walks: If possible, take a short walk after lunch. Physical activity can increase blood circulation and help prevent the post-lunch energy dip.

6. Power Nap: If you have the opportunity, consider a short power nap (around 20-30 minutes). A brief nap can refresh your mind and increase alertness without leaving you groggy.

7. Manage Stress: Practice relaxation techniques like deep breathing, meditation, or stretching exercises. Stress can drain your energy, so taking a few minutes to relax can rejuvenate your mind and body.

8. Natural Light: Spend some time outdoors or near windows to get natural light exposure. Natural light helps regulate your body's internal clock, promoting wakefulness and improving mood.

9. Limit Caffeine: While moderate caffeine intake can boost alertness, excessive amounts can lead to dehydration and disrupt your sleep patterns. Be mindful of your caffeine intake, especially in the afternoon.

10. Regular Exercise: Engage in regular physical activity. Even a short workout in the morning or during a break can improve your overall energy levels and enhance your ability to concentrate.

11. Consistent Sleep: Ensure you're getting sufficient and consistent sleep each night. Quality sleep is vital for maintaining energy levels and overall well-being.

Experiment with these strategies to find what works best for you. Everyone's body is different, so it may take some time to identify the most effective ways to manage your post-lunch energy levels.

EVENING WORKOUTS: PROS AND CONS

Here are the pros and cons of evening workouts:

Pros:

1. Increased Strength and Performance: Similar to afternoon workouts, your body temperature and muscle function tend to peak in the evening, leading to better strength and overall performance during exercises.

2. Reduced Risk of Injury: Warmer muscles and joints in the evening make your body more flexible and less prone to injuries. Proper warm-up and stretching can be more effective, lowering the risk of strains and sprains.

3. Stress Relief: Evening workouts can serve as an excellent way to unwind and relieve stress accumulated throughout the day. Physical activity triggers the release of endorphins, promoting a sense of well-being and relaxation.

4. Flexibility in Schedule: If you have a busy morning or afternoon schedule, evenings might be the only time available for your workout. This flexibility allows you to establish a consistent exercise routine.

5. Access to Facilities: Gym facilities and recreational areas are often less crowded in the evenings, providing more access to equipment and space for your workout.

6. Improved Sleep: Contrary to the belief that exercising in the evening disrupts sleep, many people find that a moderate evening workout can promote better sleep quality. However, this can vary based on individual preferences and tolerance to exercise close to bedtime.

Cons:

1. Energy Levels: After a full day of work or activities, energy levels might be lower in the evening, making it challenging to find the motivation to exercise. Fatigue can affect the quality and intensity of your workout.

2. Sleep Disruption: Intense workouts close to bedtime might disrupt sleep patterns for some individuals. It's essential to listen to your body and adjust your workout intensity and timing if you find it affects your ability to sleep restfully.

3. Evening Commitments: Social events, family responsibilities, or other evening commitments can interfere with establishing a consistent workout routine, leading to irregular exercise habits.

4. Digestion Concerns: Eating a large meal close to your workout time can cause discomfort and affect your performance. It's advisable to allow some time for digestion before engaging in intense physical activity.

5. Body Temperature Variability: While body temperature generally peaks in the evening, individual variations exist, and this peak might occur at different times for some individuals.

Ultimately, the best time for an evening workout depends on your personal preferences, energy levels, and daily schedule. Listening to your body and finding a routine that works for you is essential for maintaining a consistent and enjoyable exercise regimen.

BENEFITS OF EVENING WORKOUTS

IMPROVED ENDURANCE AND PERFORMANCE

Engaging in evening workouts offers several benefits, including improved endurance and performance. Here's how:

1. Optimal Body Temperature: In the evening, your body temperature tends to be at its highest, which can enhance muscle flexibility and reduce the risk of injuries. The increased body temperature also leads to better blood circulation, allowing your muscles to work more efficiently and improve endurance.

2. Improved Muscle Function: As your body temperature rises in the evening, your muscles become more pliable and ready for physical activity. This increased muscle flexibility and function contribute to improved endurance, allowing you to sustain exercises for longer durations without fatigue.

3. Enhanced Performance: With warmer muscles and optimal body temperature, your body is primed for physical performance. This readiness results in better strength, speed, and overall athletic performance. Whether you're running, lifting weights, or participating in sports, your body is more capable of handling the physical demands, leading to improved overall performance.

4. Effective Warm-Up: Warm-ups are crucial for preparing your body for exercise and preventing injuries. In the evening, your body is naturally warmer, making it easier and more effective to warm up your muscles and joints. A proper warm-up further enhances your endurance and performance during the main workout.

5. Better Recovery: Evening workouts can also contribute to better post-exercise recovery. After your workout, your body has the opportunity to rest and recuperate during the night, promoting muscle repair and growth. This improved recovery can lead to enhanced endurance and performance in subsequent workouts.

6. Mental Preparedness: Many people find that they are mentally prepared and motivated for evening workouts. The events of the day are over, and you can focus solely on your exercise routine. This mental readiness can translate into improved endurance, as you are more mentally engaged and committed to your workout goals.

By taking advantage of your body's natural rhythms in the evening, you can optimize your endurance and overall performance, making your workouts more effective and enjoyable. Remember to listen to your body, stay hydrated, and incorporate proper nutrition to support your fitness goals.

STRESS RELIEF AND RELAXATION

Engaging in regular physical activity, such as exercise and relaxation techniques, can provide significant stress relief and promote relaxation. Here's how:

1. Release of Endorphins: Exercise triggers the release of endorphins, often referred to as "feel-good hormones." These chemicals interact with your brain receptors, reducing your perception of pain and triggering a positive feeling in the body. This natural high can help alleviate stress and improve your mood.

2. Reduction of Cortisol: Exercise can reduce the production of cortisol, the body's stress hormone. High cortisol levels, often caused by chronic stress, can lead to various health issues. Regular physical activity helps balance cortisol levels, promoting relaxation and overall well-being.

3. Improved Sleep: Regular exercise has been linked to improved sleep quality. Getting an adequate amount of restful sleep is crucial for stress relief and relaxation. Exercise can help you fall asleep faster, deepen your sleep, and wake up feeling more refreshed.

4. Muscle Relaxation: Physical activity, especially relaxation-focused exercises like yoga and stretching, can help relax tense muscles. Stretching exercises increase blood flow to the muscles, promoting relaxation and reducing muscle tension, which is often a physical symptom of stress.

5. Mind-Body Connection: Activities like yoga and meditation emphasize the connection between the body and mind. These practices encourage mindfulness, deep breathing, and relaxation techniques, which can reduce stress, calm the mind, and enhance overall relaxation.

6. Distraction and Positive Coping: Engaging in physical activities provides a healthy distraction from daily stressors. It gives you a break from the source of stress and allows you to focus on the present moment. Exercise also provides a positive way to cope with stress, promoting a sense of control and accomplishment.

7. Social Support: Participating in group exercises or sports can provide a sense of community and social support. Interacting with others who share your interests can be uplifting and help reduce stress.

8. Improved Self-Esteem: Regular physical activity can lead to improved self-esteem and self-confidence. Achieving fitness goals, no matter how small, can boost your self-worth and provide a positive outlook on life, reducing stress in the process.

Incorporating a combination of aerobic exercises, strength training, and relaxation techniques into your routine can effectively contribute to stress relief and relaxation. It's essential to find activities that you enjoy and can sustain in the long term, making it easier to incorporate them into your daily life for ongoing stress management.

CHALLENGES OF EVENING WORKOUTS

POTENTIAL IMPACT ON SLEEP QUALITY

Engaging in evening workouts can pose challenges, particularly concerning sleep quality. Here's how evening workouts might impact your sleep and some strategies to mitigate these effects:

1. Increased Alertness: Exercise raises your body temperature and stimulates the production of hormones like adrenaline, making you more alert. For some individuals, vigorous exercise close to bedtime can make it difficult to wind down and fall asleep easily.

2. Disrupted Sleep Patterns: Intense evening workouts might disrupt your sleep cycle, making it harder to transition through the different sleep stages. Disrupted sleep patterns can lead to waking up feeling groggy or tired.

3. Delayed Bedtime: If your evening workout routine is time-consuming, it can lead to a delay in your bedtime, reducing the total amount of sleep you get, especially if you have to wake up early the next day.

4. Individual Variability: People's responses to evening exercise can vary widely. While some individuals can exercise in the evening without any impact on sleep, others may find it disruptive.

Mitigation Strategies:

1. Time Management: Schedule your workout earlier in the evening, allowing sufficient time for your body to cool down and your adrenaline levels to decrease before bedtime. Aim to finish your workout at least 2-3 hours before your intended bedtime.

2. Choose the Right Exercise: Opt for relaxation-focused activities in the evening, such as yoga, stretching, or low-intensity aerobic exercises. These activities are less likely to interfere with your sleep compared to high-intensity workouts.

3. Mindful Timing: Pay attention to your body's responses. If you notice that evening workouts consistently disrupt your sleep, consider shifting your exercise routine to earlier in the day and observe if it improves your sleep quality.

4. Establish a Bedtime Routine: Create a calming bedtime routine to help signal your body that it's time to wind down. This can include activities like reading, taking a warm bath, or practicing relaxation techniques to prepare your mind and body for sleep.

5. Monitor Caffeine Intake: Avoid consuming caffeine in the late afternoon and evening, as it can interfere with your ability to fall asleep. Caffeine is found in coffee, tea, chocolate, and some soft drinks.

6. Evaluate Individual Response: Everyone's body responds differently to exercise timing. Pay attention to your sleep patterns and adjust your workout schedule accordingly to find what works best for you.

By being mindful of the timing and intensity of your evening workouts and observing their effects on your sleep, you can make informed decisions to optimize both your fitness routine and sleep quality.

CROWDED GYM AND TIME CONSTRAINTS

Dealing with a crowded gym and time constraints can be challenging, but there are several strategies you can use to make the most out of your workout in such situations:

1. Off-Peak Hours: Try going to the gym during off-peak hours when it's less crowded. Early mornings or late evenings, especially on weekdays, are often quieter times at the gym. This can provide you with a more peaceful environment to exercise.

2. Plan Ahead: Have a well-structured workout plan before you enter the gym. Knowing exactly what exercises you need to do and in what order will help you make the most of your time. This way, you can navigate the gym efficiently, even during busy periods.

3. Superset or Circuit Workouts: Combine exercises into supersets or circuits. Supersets involve doing two exercises back-to-back with no rest in between, while circuit workouts involve performing a series of exercises in succession. These methods save time and increase the intensity of your workout.

4. Focus on Compound Exercises: Compound exercises work multiple muscle groups at once, making them more efficient. Examples include squats, deadlifts, bench presses, and pull-ups. Incorporating these exercises into your routine allows you to target several muscles in one movement, maximizing your workout efficiency.

5. Use Alternatives: If the equipment you need is occupied, be open to using alternative machines or free weights that target the same muscle group. Being flexible with your workout routine ensures you can adapt to the gym's busy environment.

6. HIIT Workouts: High-Intensity Interval Training (HIIT) involves short bursts of intense exercise followed by brief periods of rest. HIIT workouts are time-efficient and can be adapted to various exercises, providing an effective workout in a limited timeframe.

7. Home Workouts: Consider incorporating home workouts into your routine, especially on days when you have time constraints or the gym is exceptionally crowded. There are numerous bodyweight exercises and home workout routines available online that require minimal equipment.

8. Be Patient and Flexible: Sometimes, you might need to wait for a specific piece of equipment. Use this time to perform other exercises or stretches. Being patient and adaptable can help you stay focused and make the most of your gym session.

Remember, consistency is key to progress in your fitness journey. Even if you have limited time or face a crowded gym, making the most of the resources available and staying committed to your workout routine can lead to significant improvements in your fitness levels.

TAILORING THE WORKOUT TIME TO INDIVIDUAL GOALS

Designing a workout routine tailored to individual goals is a personalized approach that maximizes efficiency and effectiveness. By understanding your specific objectives, you can optimize your fitness plan to achieve desired results. Whether you aim to build muscle, improve endurance, lose weight, or enhance flexibility, tailoring your workout time to your goals is essential for success.

In this personalized approach, various factors come into play, including the type of exercises, workout intensity, duration, and frequency. By customizing these elements to align with your fitness goals, you can create a targeted and efficient workout routine. Let's explore how adjusting these aspects can address specific fitness objectives, providing a clear path toward achieving your goals.

WEIGHT LOSS AND FAT BURNING

When the goal is weight loss and fat burning, tailoring your workout routine becomes crucial. Here's how you can design an effective fitness plan to achieve these objectives:

1. Cardiovascular Exercises: Cardio workouts, such as running, cycling, swimming, and aerobics, are excellent for burning calories and promoting fat loss. Aim for at least 150 minutes of moderate-intensity aerobic exercise or 75 minutes of vigorous-intensity aerobic exercise per week, as recommended by health authorities.

2. High-Intensity Interval Training (HIIT): HIIT involves short bursts of intense exercise followed by brief periods of rest or low-intensity activity. This approach can significantly boost your metabolism, increase fat burning, and improve cardiovascular fitness in a shorter amount of time. HIIT workouts can include activities like sprinting, jumping jacks, or cycling at maximum effort for short intervals.

3. Strength Training: Incorporate resistance training exercises using weights, resistance bands, or body weight. Building lean muscle mass not only improves your metabolism but also contributes to a toned appearance. Include compound exercises like squats, lunges, push-ups, and deadlifts, targeting major muscle groups to maximize calorie burn.

4. Flexibility and Mobility Exercises: While not directly burning a significant number of calories, stretching and flexibility exercises (e.g., yoga, Pilates) are essential for injury prevention and overall well-being. They can be included in your routine to enhance your range of motion and make other workouts more effective.

5. Consistency and Progression: Stay consistent with your workouts and gradually increase the intensity and duration over time. As your fitness level improves, challenge yourself with more advanced exercises and longer workout sessions to continue burning fat and losing weight.

6. Balanced Diet: Remember that exercise is just one part of the equation. Pair your workouts with a balanced, calorie-controlled diet rich in whole foods, lean proteins, fruits, vegetables, and whole grains. Proper nutrition is essential for weight loss and overall health.

7. Adequate Rest and Recovery: Allow your body to rest and recover to prevent burnout and injuries. Aim for 7-9 hours of quality sleep each night, as sleep plays a vital role in regulating hormones related to hunger and metabolism.

By combining cardiovascular exercises, HIIT, strength training, flexibility work, a balanced diet, and sufficient rest, you can create a comprehensive fitness plan tailored to promote weight loss and fat burning. Remember that consistency and dedication to your goals are key to achieving lasting results.

OPTIMAL TIMING FOR CALORIE BURN

The optimal timing for calorie burn largely depends on your personal schedule, preferences, and lifestyle. Here are a few factors to consider when deciding the best time to focus on calorie burn through exercise:

1. Morning Workouts: Exercising in the morning can boost your metabolism early in the day, setting a positive tone for the rest of the day. Some studies suggest that morning workouts may help you burn

more calories throughout the day due to the "afterburn effect" (excess post-exercise oxygen consumption). Additionally, morning exercise can enhance mental alertness and productivity.

2. Afternoon and Evening Workouts: Exercising in the afternoon or evening can take advantage of your body's increased temperature and improved muscle function during these times. This can lead to better performance and calorie burn during workouts. Evening workouts can also serve as a stress reliever after a busy day.

3. Consistency Matters: The best time to burn calories is when you can be consistent with your workout routine. Regular exercise, regardless of the time of day, contributes significantly to your overall calorie burn and fitness level. Consistency and adherence to your exercise regimen are more important than the specific time you choose to work out.

4. Personal Preference: Some people are naturally more energetic and motivated in the morning, while others feel more alert and capable in the afternoon or evening. Choose a time that aligns with your natural energy levels and makes it easier for you to stay committed to your fitness goals.

5. Avoid Late-Night Workouts: Exercising very close to bedtime might disrupt your sleep patterns for some individuals. It's generally advisable to finish intense workouts at least 2-3 hours before bedtime to allow your body to wind down and prepare for rest.

Ultimately, the best time for calorie burn is when you can consistently engage in physical activity. Whether it's morning, afternoon, or evening, the key is to find a time that fits your schedule, energy levels, and personal preferences. Regular exercise, combined with a balanced diet and proper rest, is essential for overall health and effective calorie burn.

INCORPORATING HIGH INTENSITY INTERVAL TRAINING

Incorporating High-Intensity Interval Training (HIIT) into your fitness routine can be an efficient and effective way to burn calories, improve cardiovascular health, and increase overall fitness. Here's how you can integrate HIIT workouts into your regimen:

1. Start with a Warm-Up: Begin your HIIT session with a 5-10 minute warm-up. Engage in light cardio exercises like jogging, jumping jacks, or cycling to increase your heart rate and prepare your muscles for the intense workout ahead.

2. Choose Your Exercises: Select a set of exercises that target different muscle groups. Bodyweight exercises like squats, push-ups, lunges, burpees, and mountain climbers are excellent choices. You can also incorporate cardio exercises like sprinting, jumping rope, or cycling.

3. Set Interval Times: Structure your HIIT workout into intervals of high-intensity exercise followed by periods of rest or low-intensity activity. For example, work hard for 30 seconds and then rest or perform low-intensity exercise for 30 seconds to 1 minute. Repeat this cycle for a specific number of rounds, usually ranging from 4 to 8, depending on your fitness level.

4. Increase Intensity: During the high-intensity intervals, give it your all. Push yourself to work at maximum effort, whether it's doing exercises as fast as possible, increasing resistance, or adding explosive movements. The intensity is what makes HIIT effective.

5. Stay Consistent: Consistency is key to seeing results with HIIT. Aim to incorporate HIIT workouts into your routine 2-3 times per week. As you progress, you can gradually increase the duration of your HIIT sessions or the intensity of the exercises.

6. Include a Cool Down: After completing your high-intensity intervals, spend 5-10 minutes cooling down. Perform stretches to relax your muscles and improve flexibility. This helps prevent muscle soreness and promotes recovery.

7. Listen to Your Body: HIIT is challenging, so it's essential to listen to your body. If you're a beginner, start with shorter intervals and lower intensity, then gradually increase as your fitness level improves. If you have any health concerns or injuries, consult a fitness professional or healthcare provider before starting HIIT.

8. Combine with Other Workouts: You can integrate HIIT into your existing workout routine. For example, you might do HIIT on alternate days while focusing on strength training or endurance exercises on other days. This combination provides a well-rounded approach to fitness.

Remember, HIIT can be adapted to various fitness levels and can be done with minimal or no equipment. It offers a time-efficient way to burn calories, making it an excellent addition to your fitness arsenal.

MUSCLE BUILDING AND STRENGHT TRAINING

Building muscle and improving strength require a combination of targeted exercises, proper nutrition, and adequate rest and recovery. Here's how you can tailor your workout routine for muscle building and strength training:

1. Focus on Compound Exercises: Compound exercises work multiple muscle groups at once, making them highly effective for building overall muscle mass and strength. Include exercises like squats, deadlifts, bench presses, pull-ups, and rows in your routine. These exercises engage large muscle groups and promote significant muscle growth.

2. Progressive Overload: To build muscle and strength, gradually increase the weight or resistance you use in your exercises over time. Progressive overload challenges your muscles, forcing them to adapt and grow stronger. Aim to increase the weight or resistance when you can perform the current weight comfortably for the recommended sets and repetitions.

3. Lift Heavy Weights: Use challenging weights that allow you to perform 6-12 repetitions with proper form. This rep range is generally considered optimal for muscle hypertrophy (growth). Lifting heavy weights with proper technique stimulates muscle fibers, promoting muscle development.

4. Include Isolation Exercises: While compound exercises are essential, isolation exercises target specific muscle groups. Include exercises like bicep curls, triceps extensions, calf raises, and leg curls to focus on individual muscles. Isolation exercises help sculpt and define specific muscle groups.

5. Rest and Recovery: Muscles need time to recover and grow stronger after intense workouts. Ensure you get adequate sleep (7-9 hours per night) and allow at least 48 hours of rest between working the same muscle group. This recovery time is crucial for muscle repair and growth.

6. Nutrition: Consume a balanced diet with a focus on protein, which is essential for muscle repair and growth. Include sources of lean protein such as chicken, fish, tofu, beans, and dairy products in your meals. Also, ensure you're getting enough carbohydrates for energy and healthy fats for overall well-being.

7. Stay Hydrated: Proper hydration is crucial for muscle function and overall performance. Drink water throughout the day, especially during and after your workouts, to stay properly hydrated.

8. Consistency: Consistency is key in muscle building and strength training. Stick to your workout routine and be patient. Building muscle takes time and dedication. Track your progress, celebrate your achievements, and adjust your routine as needed to keep challenging your muscles.

9. Proper Form: Maintain proper form during exercises to prevent injuries and effectively target the intended muscles. If you're unsure about the correct technique, consider working with a certified personal trainer who can guide you.

By incorporating these principles into your strength training routine, you can effectively build muscle, increase strength, and achieve your fitness goals. Remember that individual responses to training may vary, so it's essential to find an approach that works best for your body and fitness level.

TIMING PROTEIN INTAKE AND WORKOUTS

Timing your protein intake around your workouts can significantly impact muscle recovery and growth. Here are some guidelines on when to consume protein concerning your workout schedule:

1. Before Workouts:

   Pre-Workout Meal (1-3 hours before): Include a balance of protein and carbohydrates in your pre-workout meal. This combination provides sustained energy and ensures that your body has amino acids available for muscle preservation and repair during exercise.

2. During Workouts (for Endurance Athletes):

   Long-duration Workouts: Endurance athletes engaging in prolonged activities (such as marathon running or cycling) might benefit from consuming easily digestible protein and carbohydrates during extended workouts. Protein sources like protein bars or shakes can provide amino acids to prevent muscle breakdown during long, intense sessions.

3. After Workouts:

   Post-Workout Nutrition (within 30 minutes to 1 hour after): Consuming protein and carbohydrates shortly after your workout is crucial for muscle recovery and replenishing glycogen stores. A protein-rich snack or shake combined with carbohydrates helps kick-start the muscle repair process and refuels energy stores.

CONCLUSION

Here's a recap of the key points regarding workout timing:

1. Morning Workouts:

   - Boost metabolism early in the day.

   - Enhance mental alertness and productivity.

   - Good for establishing a routine.

2. Afternoon/Evening Workouts:

   - Benefit from increased body temperature and muscle function.

   - Improve strength and endurance due to optimal body conditions.

   - Serve as stress relief after a busy day.

3. Nutrition and Hydration:

   - Have a balanced meal 1-3 hours before exercising.

   - Consume protein and carbohydrates after workouts for muscle recovery.

   - Stay hydrated throughout the day, especially before, during, and after exercise.

4. High-Intensity Interval Training (HIIT):

   - Incorporate HIIT for efficient calorie burn and improved cardiovascular health.

   - Ideal for shorter, intense workouts and time-efficient training.

5. Muscle Building and Strength Training:

   - Focus on compound exercises to target multiple muscle groups.

   - Lift heavy weights with proper form for muscle hypertrophy.

   - Prioritize protein intake for muscle repair and growth.

6. Consistency and Recovery:

   - Consistency is key for progress; make exercise a habit.

   - Plan rest days to prevent injuries and allow muscles to recover.

   - Listen to your body, adjust routines, and prioritize sleep and nutrition for optimal recovery.

Remember, individual preferences, energy levels, and schedules play a significant role in determining the best workout time. It's essential to find a routine that aligns with your lifestyle and allows for consistent, enjoyable, and effective workouts. Always consult with a healthcare provider or fitness professional if you have specific health concerns or goals.

EMPHASIZING THE SIGNIFICANCE OF FINDING THE BEST TIME BASED ON INDIVIDUAL PREFERENCES AND SCHEDULES

Emphasizing the significance of finding the best workout time based on individual preferences and schedules is crucial for establishing a sustainable and effective fitness routine. Here's why personalized timing matters:

1. Consistency and Adherence: Choosing a workout time that aligns with your natural energy levels and daily schedule increases the likelihood of sticking to your fitness routine. Consistency is key to achieving long-term fitness goals.

2. Optimal Performance: Exercising at a time when you feel most energetic and motivated enhances your overall performance. You're more likely to push yourself, leading to better results and a sense of accomplishment.

3. Reduced Stress: A workout time that fits seamlessly into your daily routine reduces stress associated with time constraints and conflicting schedules. It allows you to approach exercise with a relaxed mindset, enhancing the overall experience.

4. Improved Mood and Enjoyment: Exercising at a time that suits you best enhances your mood and enjoyment during workouts. When you enjoy your exercise routine, you're more likely to look forward to it, making it a positive part of your day.

5. Better Sleep and Recovery: For some individuals, evening workouts might interfere with sleep, while others find them relaxing. By understanding your body's response to exercise timing, you can ensure that your workouts support, rather than disrupt, your sleep and recovery patterns.

6. Flexibility and Adaptability: Life is dynamic, and schedules can change. Finding a workout time that aligns with your preferences allows for flexibility. You can adjust your routine to accommodate changes in your daily life without disrupting your fitness habits.

7. Customized Approach: Every person is unique, and what works best for one individual might not suit another. By considering your own preferences, energy levels, and lifestyle, you can tailor your fitness routine to meet your specific needs and goals.

In summary, the best workout time is the one that fits seamlessly into your life, energizes you, and makes exercising a positive and sustainable experience. By listening to your body and aligning your workouts with your individual preferences and schedules, you can create a fitness routine that becomes an integral and enjoyable part of your daily life.

ENCOURAGEMENTS FOR READERS TO ESTABLISH A CONSISTENT WORKOUT ROUTINE REGARDLESS OF THE TIME OF DAY

Establishing a consistent workout routine, regardless of the time of day, is a powerful commitment to your well-being and long-term health. Here's some encouragement for you:

Remember, every step you take toward a healthier lifestyle is a victory. Whether you're a morning person, prefer midday workouts, or thrive in the evening, the key is consistency. Regular exercise is not just about physical transformation; it's about the journey of becoming your best self, inside and out.

Embrace the time that works for you, considering your schedule and energy levels. The important thing is to find a routine that you enjoy and can sustain. Your commitment to consistent workouts is a testament to your dedication, discipline, and self-care.

With every workout, you're investing in your future health, building strength, resilience, and confidence. Celebrate your progress, no matter how small it might seem, because each step forward is a step toward a healthier, happier you.

Stay persistent, stay motivated, and most importantly, be kind to yourself. Every effort you put in counts, and over time, those efforts add up to significant, positive changes in your life. Your consistent dedication to your fitness journey is a source of inspiration, not only for yourself but also for those around you.

So, lace up those shoes, hit the gym, go for that run, or roll out your yoga mat. Regardless of the time of day, every workout brings you closer to your dream.